THE
ULTIMATE
BULLWORKER

POWER REP RANGE

WORKOUTS

The ULTIMATE BULLWORKER POWER REP RANGE

WORKOUTS

The Best Isotonic/Isometric Exercises to build muscle, increase strength, burn fat and sculpt the best body with the power of Rep Range and Isometrics!

BECOME A RIPPED BULLWORKER MAN!

The Ultimate Bullworker Power Rep Range Workouts was written to help you get closer to your physical potential when it comes to real muscle sculpting strengthening exercises. The exercises and routines in this book are quite demanding, so consult your physician and have a physical exam taken prior to the start of this exercise program. Proceed with the suggested exercises and information at your own risk. The Publishers and author shall not be liable or responsible for any loss, injury, or damage allegedly arising from the information or suggestions in this book.

The Ultimate Bullworker Power Rep Range Workouts
muscle-building program

By

Birch Tree Publishing
Published by Birch Tree Publishing

The Ultimate Bullworker Power Rep Range Workouts
published in 2019, All rights reserved,

© 2019 Copyright Birch Tree Publishing
Brought to you by the
Publishers of Birch Tree Publishing
ISBN-978-1-927558-86-7

Birch Tree Publishing

Dedication

Become Transformed **TODAY!**

Contents

Finally "GET" TRANSFORMED

with the, Power Rep Range Workouts
the fastest muscle-producing program
right in the palms of your hands!

Introduction by Marlon Birch CSCS

Trainees of our "Bullworker Power Series" know that we present the best muscle-building programs to increase optimum strength and add quality to one's life. That's our goal at Bullworker.

This book introduces The Bullworker Power Rep Range Workouts these programs will get you in the best shape **FASTER** than you thought possible. With the power of our system- and the muscle-building benefits of isometrics holds. Combining Isotonics and Isometrics forces the muscles to contract harder and over come neuromuscular system failure.

Our methods extend a set beyond failure, and you will see muscle popping up almost overnight. While getting more muscular and leaner than ever before. It's an eye-opening program that can help you pack on muscle and strength fast. We also look at the optimal rep speed for you to keep building muscles while applying various factors to increase growth.

Keep moving forward

Marlon Birch
Yours In Health and Strength

FULL-BODY WORKOUTS

CHAPTER 1
STANDARD PROGRAM
PHASE ONE
2 WEEKS
REP SPEED CONTRACT 1 SECOND, RELEASE 1 SECOND

01 STANDARD PROGRAM PHASE ONE

Perform 10 full reps, followed by 10 half reps. At the start position to the mid-point of the exercise stroke. On the 10th half rep perform a 20 second Isometric contraction. Two sets each exercise. All exercises are done non stop until one round is finished. Rest 5 seconds between rounds. Alternate day one and day two for 6 days per week.

DAY ONE

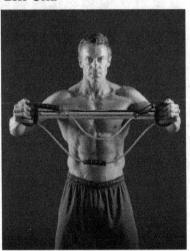
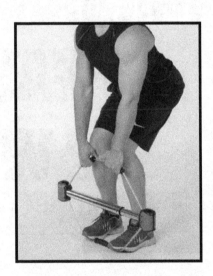
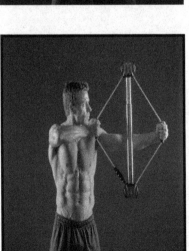
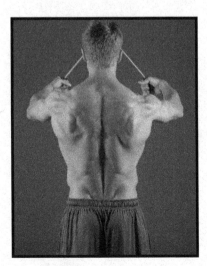

01 STANDARD PROGRAM PHASE ONE

DAY ONE CONTINUED.....

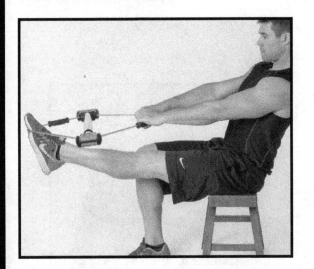
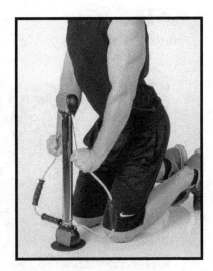

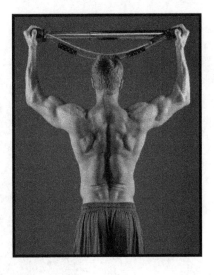
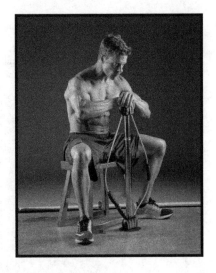

01 STANDARD PROGRAM

DAY TWO
Same instructions as Day one.

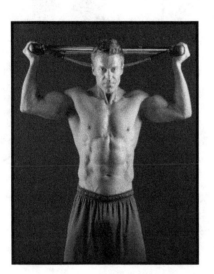

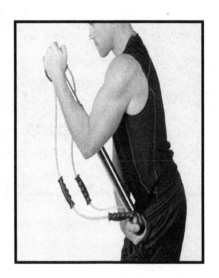

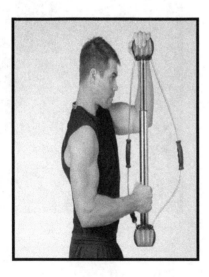

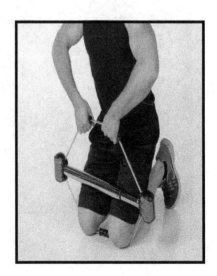

01 STANDARD PROGRAM
DAY TWO CONTINUED.......

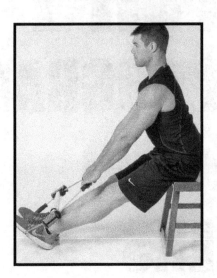

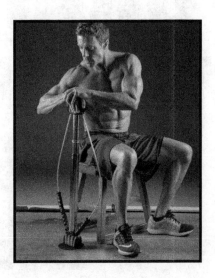

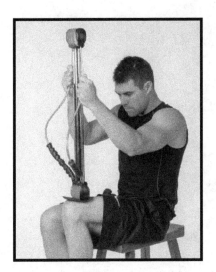

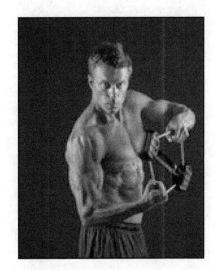

CHAPTER 1
STANDARD PROGRAM
PHASE TWO
2 WEEKS
REP SPEED CONTRACT 1 SECOND, RELEASE 1 SECOND

01 STANDARD PROGRAM

Perform 15 full reps, followed by 15 half reps. At the start position to the mid-point of the exercise stroke. On the 15th half rep perform a 10 second Isometric contraction. Three sets each exercise. All exercises are done non stop until one round is finished. Rest 5 seconds between rounds. Alternate day one and day two for 6 days per week.

DAY ONE

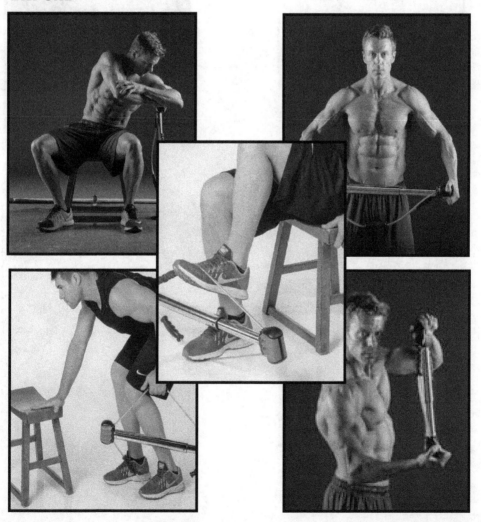

01 STANDARD PROGRAM

DAY TWO

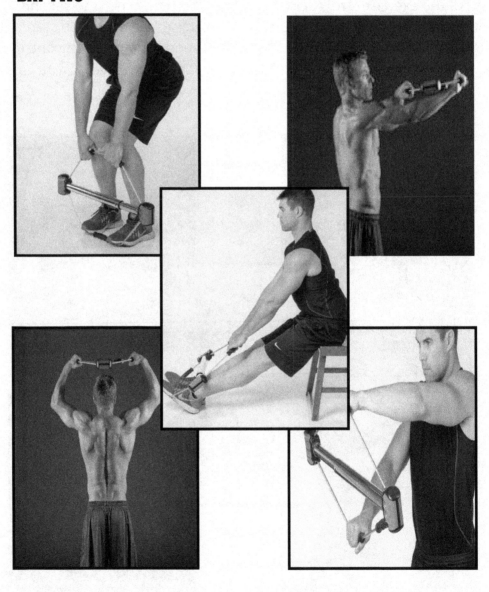

CHAPTER 2
POWER SURGE

PHASE THREE

3 WEEKS
REP SPEED CONTRACT 1 SECOND, RELEASE 3 SECONDS

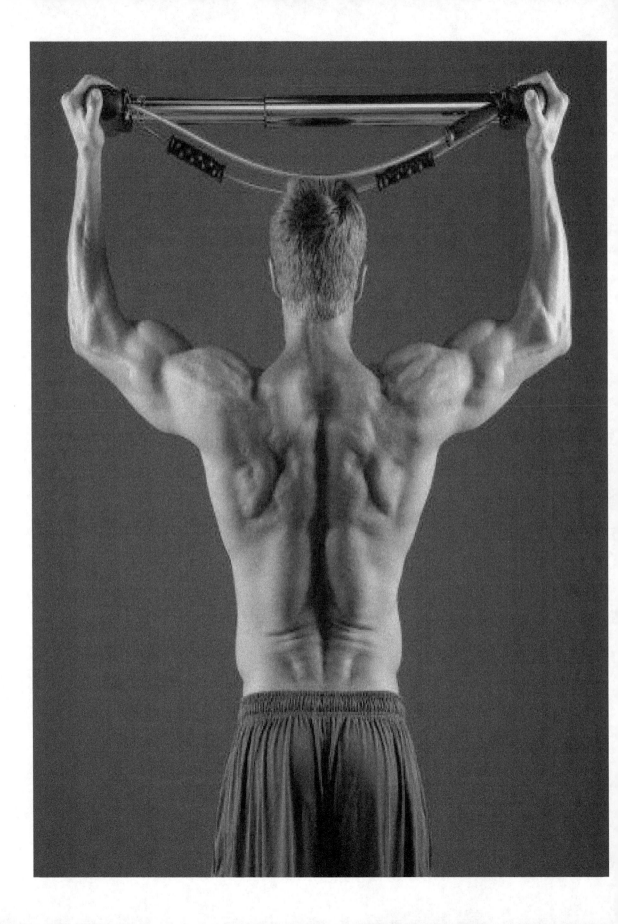

02 POWER SURGE PROGRAM

Perform all exercises non-stop. No isometric hold or half reps within this phase.
Perform 7-9 reps per bodypart at 4 sets each.

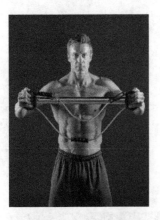
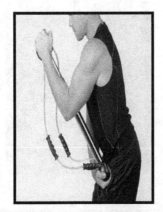
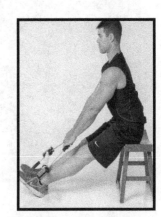

MON, WED, FRI

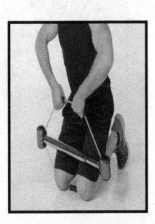
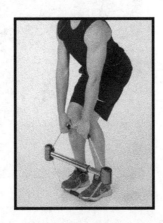
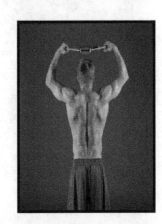

02 POWER SURGE PROGRAM

Perform all exercises non-stop. No isometric hold or half reps within this phase. Perform 5-7 reps per bodypart at 4-5 sets each.

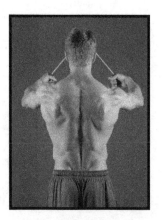
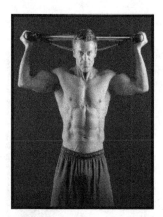
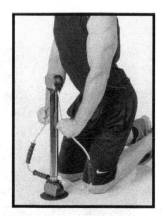

TUES, THURS, SAT

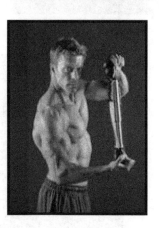
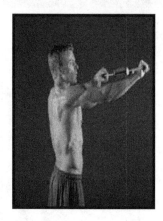
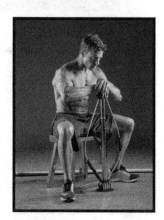

CHAPTER 2
POWER SURGE
PHASE FOUR
3 WEEKS
REP SPEED CONTRACT 1 SECOND, RELEASE 3 SECONDS

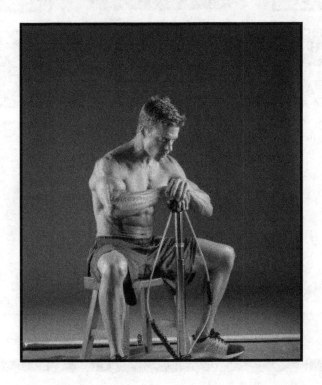

02 POWER SURGE PROGRAM

Perform 7-9 full reps, followed by 10 half reps. At the start position to the mid-point of the exercise stroke. On the 10th half rep perform a 20 second Isometric contraction. Three sets each exercise. All exercises are done non stop until one round is finished. Rest 5 seconds between rounds.

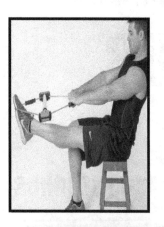
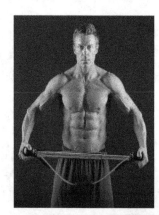
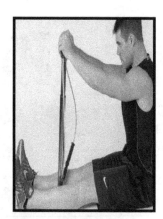

MON, WED, FRI

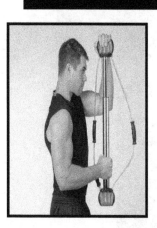
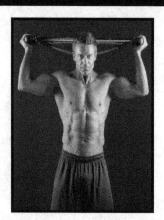
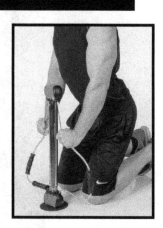

02 POWER SURGE PROGRAM

Perform 7-9 full reps, followed by 10 half reps. At the start position to the mid-point of the exercise stroke. On the 10th half rep perform a 20 second Isometric contraction. Three sets each exercise. All exercises are done non stop until one round is finished. Rest 5 seconds between rounds.

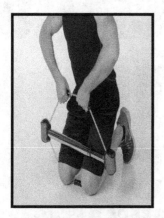
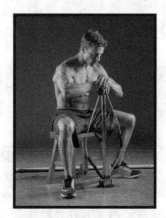
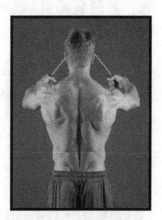

TUES, THURS, SAT

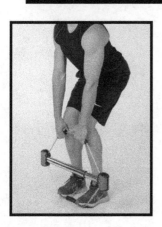
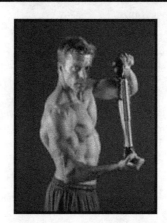
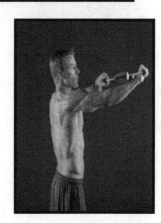

CHAPTER 3
SUPERCOMPENSATION
PHASE FIVE
3 WEEKS

REP SPEED CONTRACT 2 SECONDS, RELEASE 6 SECONDS

03 SUPERCOMPENSATION PROGRAM

Perform a 10 second Isometric contraction, followed by 5 reps. On the 5th rep perform 15 half reps from the start position to mid-point then hold for a 20 second contraction. Perform all exercises non-stop until one full round is completed. Rest 5 seconds and complete a total of 4 rounds.

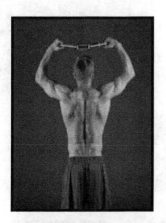
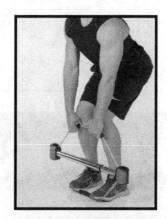
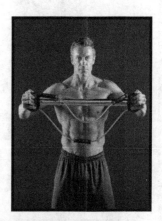

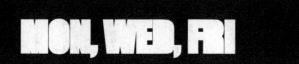

MON, WED, FRI

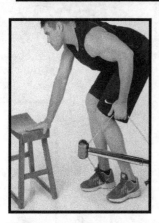
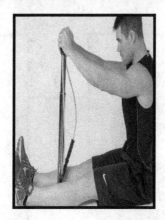
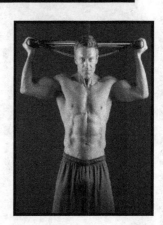

03 SUPERCOMPENSATION PROGRAM

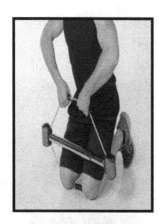 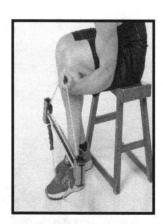 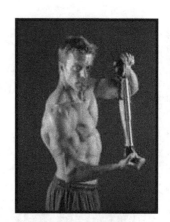

TUES, THURS, SAT

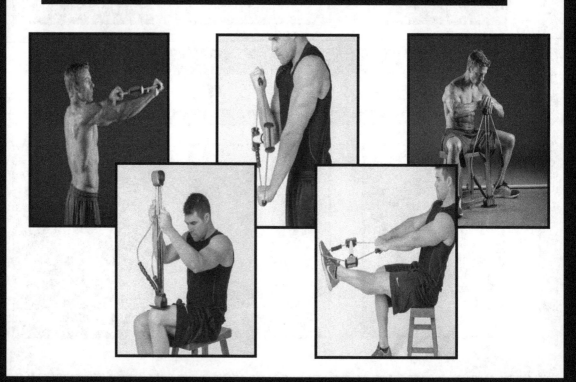

CHAPTER 3
SUPERCOMPENSATION
PHASE SIX
3 WEEKS
REP SPEED CONTRACT 1 SECOND, RELEASE 1 SECOND

03 SUPERCOMPENSATION PROGRAM

Perform a 20 second Isometric contraction, followed by 15 reps. On the 15th rep perform 10 half reps from the start position to mid-point then hold for a 30 second contraction. Perform all exercises non-stop until one full round is completed. Rest 5 seconds and complete a total of 3 rounds.

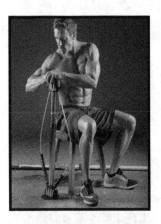
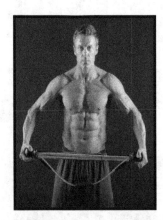
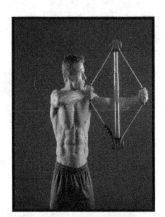

MON, WED, FRI

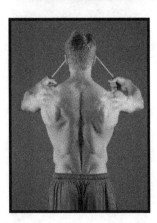
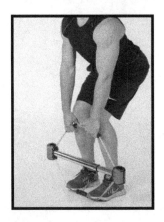
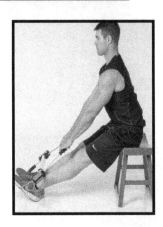

03 SUPERCOMPENSATION PROGRAM

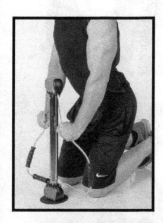
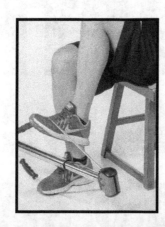
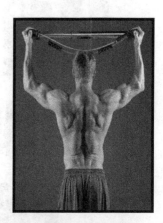

TUES, THURS, SAT

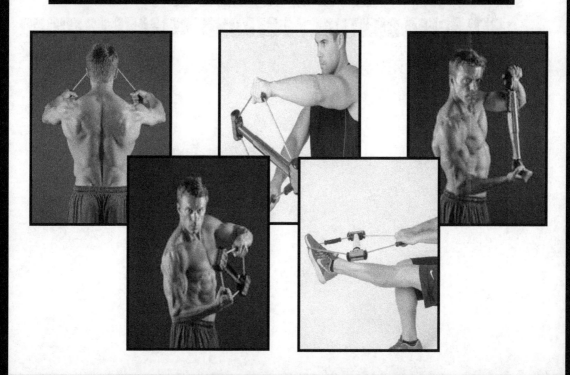

CHAPTER 4
POWER PYRAMID
PHASE SEVEN
2 WEEKS
REP SPEED CONTRACT 1 SECOND, RELEASE 1 SECOND

04 POWER PYRAMID PROGRAM

On each exercise perform 10,8,7,6 reps. At the end of each rep range perform a 10 second isometric contraction. Continue until all bodyparts are completed. Perform 2 rounds in total.

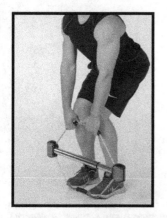
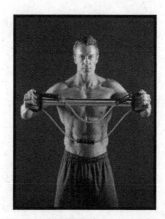
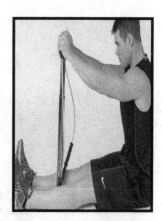

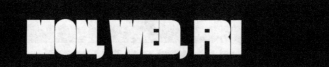

MON, WED, FRI

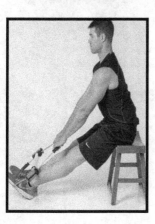
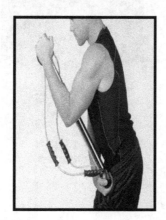
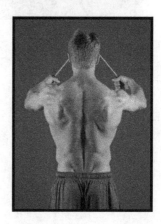

04 POWER PYRAMID PROGRAM

On each exercise perform 15, 10, 8 reps. At the end of each rep range perform a 10 second isometric contraction. Continue until all bodyparts are completed. Perform 3 rounds in total.

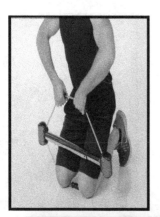
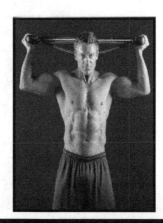
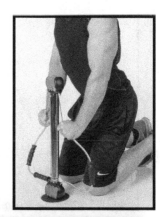

TUES, THURS, SAT

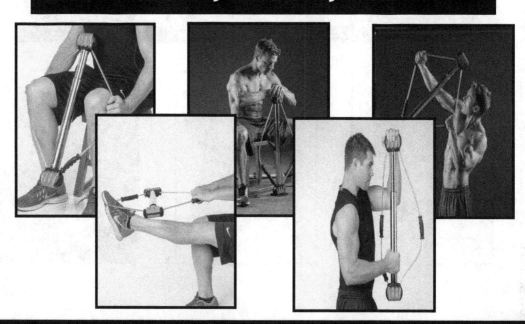

CHAPTER 5
POWER MAX 20/20/20
PHASE EIGHT
2 WEEKS
REP SPEED CONTRACT 1 SECOND, RELEASE 1 SECOND

POWER MAX 20/20/20 PROGRAM

05 POWER MAX PROGRAM 20,20,20   DAY ONE

HOW TO PERFORM THIS ROUTINE: Perform 20 reps, followed by an isometric contraction for 20 seconds, without rest perform a final 20 reps.
PERFORM THREE ROUNDS (SETS)

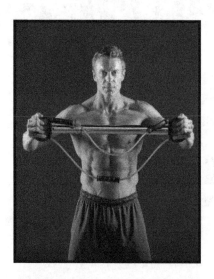
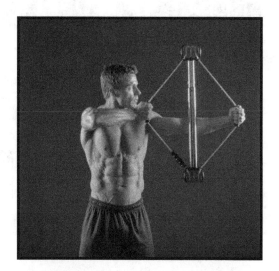
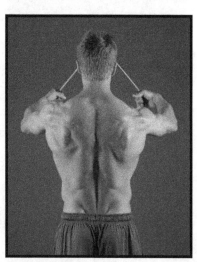
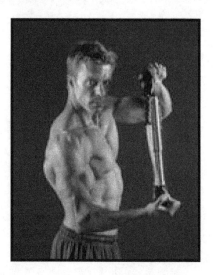

POWER MAX 20/20/20 PROGRAM

05 POWER MAX PROGRAM 20,20,20 DAY TWO

HOW TO PERFORM THIS ROUTINE: Perform 20 reps, followed by an isometric contraction for 20 seconds, without rest perform a final 20 reps.
PERFORM THREE ROUNDS (SETS)

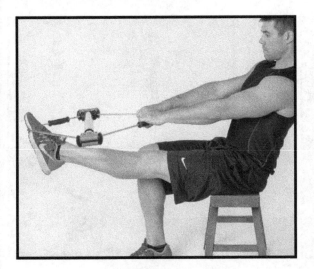
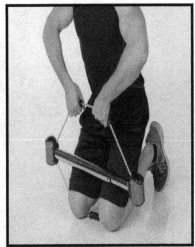
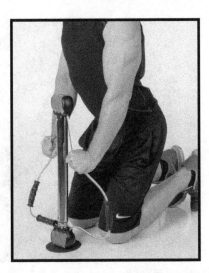
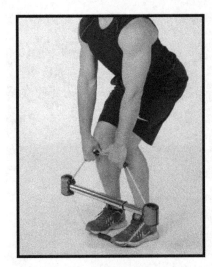

POWER MAX 20/20/20 PROGRAM

05 POWER MAX PROGRAM 20,20,20 DAY THREE

HOW TO PERFORM THIS ROUTINE: Perform 20 reps, followed by an isometric contraction for 20 seconds, without rest perform a final 20 reps.
PERFORM THREE ROUNDS (SETS)

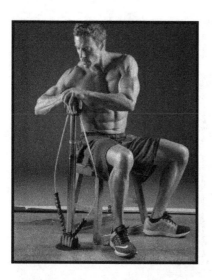
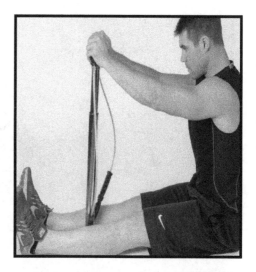
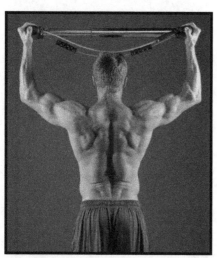
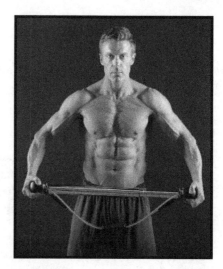

POWER MAX 20/20/20 PROGRAM

05 POWER MAX PROGRAM 20,20,20 DAY FOUR

HOW TO PERFORM THIS ROUTINE: Perform 20 reps, followed by an isometric contraction for 20 seconds, without rest perform a final 20 reps.
PERFORM THREE ROUNDS (SETS)

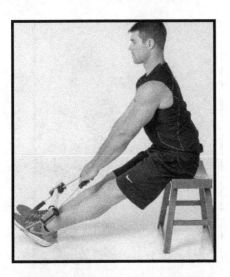
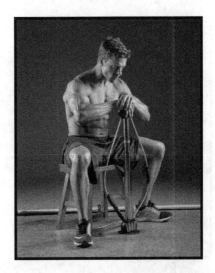
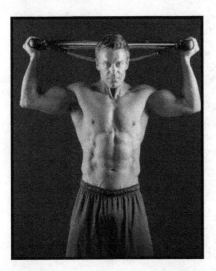
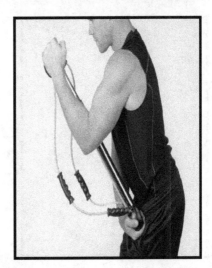

POWER MAX 20/20/20 PROGRAM

05 POWER MAX PROGRAM 20,20,20 DAY FIVE

HOW TO PERFORM THIS ROUTINE: Perform 20 reps, followed by an isometric contraction for 20 seconds, without rest perform a final 20 reps.
PERFORM THREE ROUNDS (SETS)

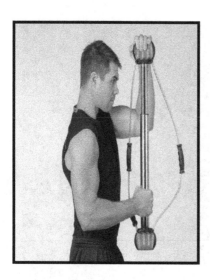
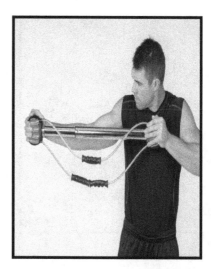
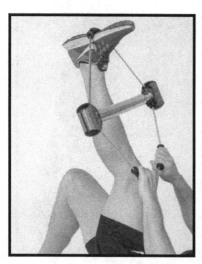
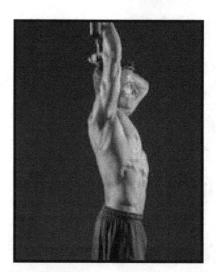

POWER FIVE PROGRAM

06 POWER FIVE STRENGTH PROGRAM

MONDAY, WEDNESDAY, FRIDAY
HOW TO PERFORM THIS ROUTINE: You contract for 2 seconds and release for a slow 6 seconds. Perform 5 reps; each rep perform an isometric contraction for 5 seconds. Perform 3 rounds.
Perform plan for 2 weeks before moving to Phase Ten.

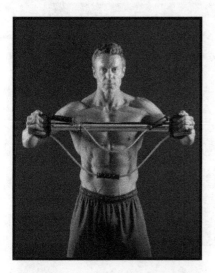
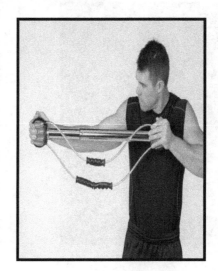
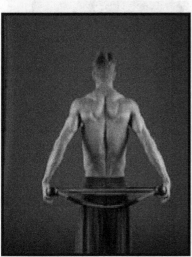
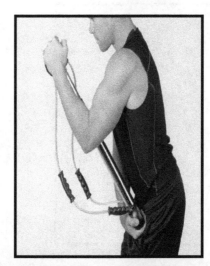

POWER FIVE PROGRAM

06 POWER FIVE STRENGTH PROGRAM

MONDAY,WEDNESDAY,FRIDAY
Routine continued.............

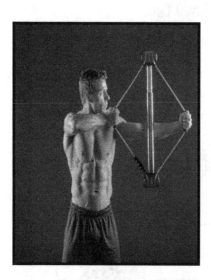

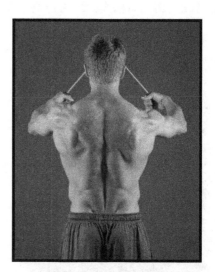

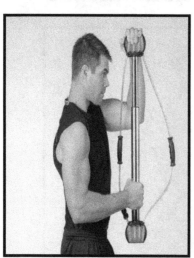

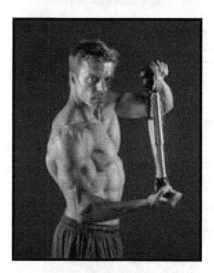

POWER FIVE PROGRAM

06 POWER FIVE STRENGTH PROGRAM

MONDAY, WEDNESDAY, FRIDAY
Routine continued.............

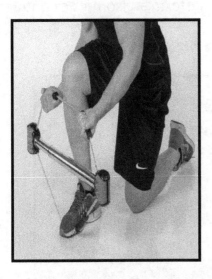 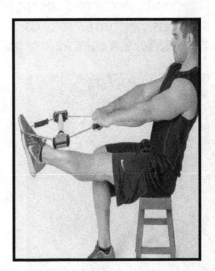

PHASE NINE MON, WED, FRI

POWER FIVE PROGRAM

06 POWER FIVE STRENGTH PROGRAM

TUESDAY, THURSDAY, SATURDAY
HOW TO PERFORM THIS ROUTINE: You contract for 2 seconds and release for a slow 6 seconds. Perform 5 reps; each rep perform an isometric contraction for 5 seconds. Perform 3 rounds.
Perform plan for 2 weeks before moving to Phase Ten.

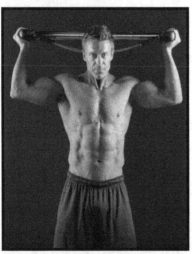

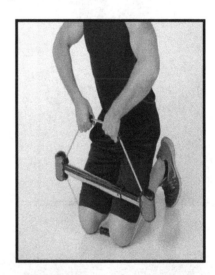

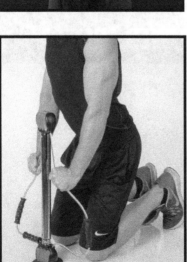

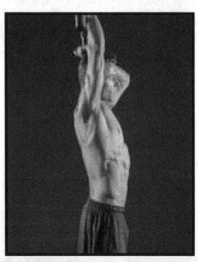

POWER FIVE PROGRAM

06 POWER FIVE STRENGTH PROGRAM

TUESDAY, THURSDAY, SATURDAY
Routine continued...................

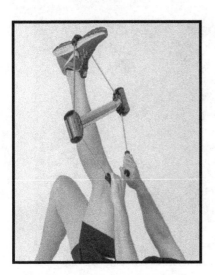
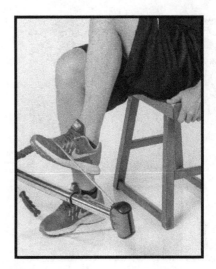

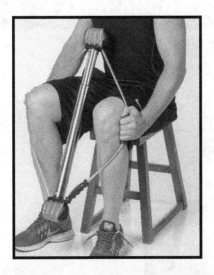
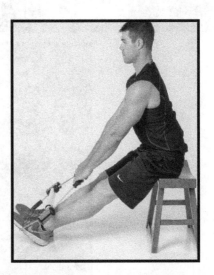

POWER FIVE PROGRAM

06 POWER FIVE STRENGTH PROGRAM

TUESDAY, THURSDAY, SATURDAY
Routine continued...................

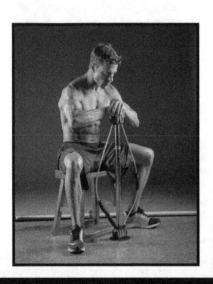 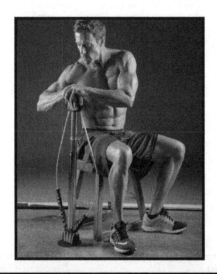

PHASE NINE TUES, THURS, SAT.

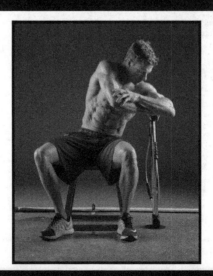

DENSITY REP RANGE

07 DENSITY REP RANGE PROGRAM 15,10,7

MONDAY, WEDNESDAY, FRIDAY
HOW TO PERFORM THIS ROUTINE: You contract within 1 second and release 1 second. Perform 15 reps followed by a 5 second isometric, 10 reps followed by another 5 second isometric, then a final 7 reps. On the 7th rep hold for a 20 second Isometric contraction. **Perform program for 2 weeks**

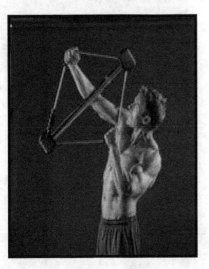
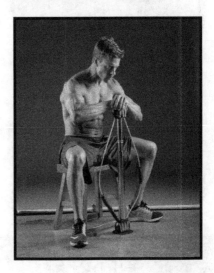
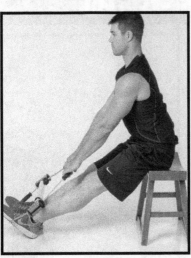
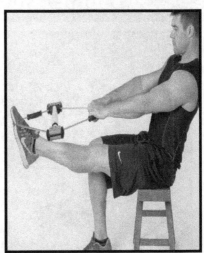

DENSITY REP RANGE

07 DENSITY REP RANGE PROGRAM 15,10,7

MONDAY, WEDNESDAY, FRIDAY
Routine continued............

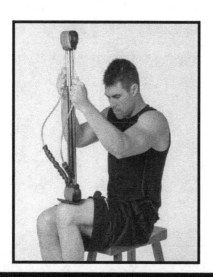 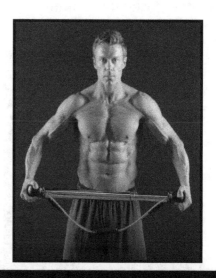

PHASE TEN   MON, WED, FRI.

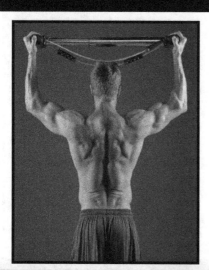 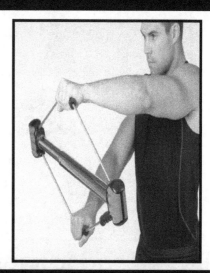

DENSITY REP RANGE

07 DENSITY REP RANGE PROGRAM 7,5,7

TUESDAY, THURSDAY, SATURDAY

You contract within 1 second and slowly release the tension for 3 seconds. Perform 7 reps followed by a 5 second isometric, 5 reps followed by another 5 second isometric, then a final 7 reps. On the 7th rep hold for a 20 second Isometric contraction.

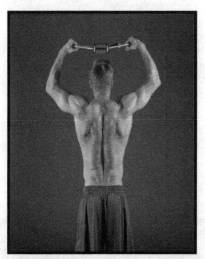
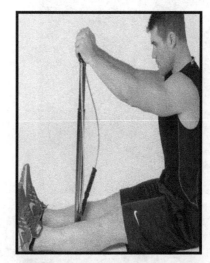
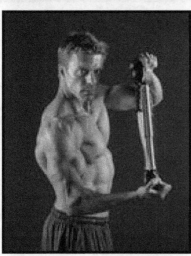
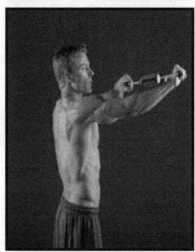

DENSITY REP RANGE

07 DENSITY REP RANGE PROGRAM 7,5,7

TUESDAY, THURSDAY, SATURDAY
Routine continued...................

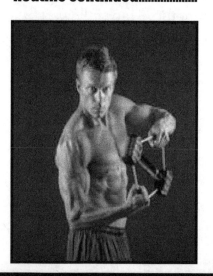

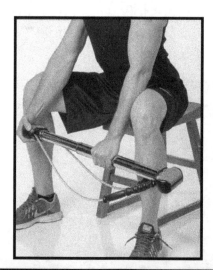

PHASE TEN   TUES, THURS, SAT.

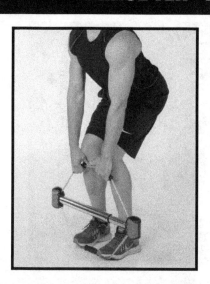

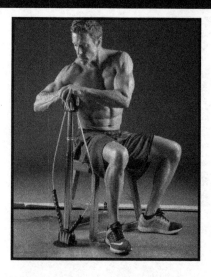

CHAPTER 8
REP RANGE 20/10/30
PHASE 11
3 WEEKS

REP SPEED CONTRACT 1 SECOND, RELEASE 1 SECOND
FIRST WEEK 20 REPS, 20 SECOND ISOMETRIC... 3 ROUNDS
SECOND WEEK 10 REPS, 10 SECOND ISOMETRIC.. 3 ROUNDS
THIRD WEEK 30 REPS, 30 SECOND ISOMETRIC... 2 ROUNDS

REP RANGE 20,10,30

08 REP RANGE PROGRAM

HOW TO PERFORM THIS ROUTINE:
First Week Perform 20 reps, 20 second Isometric contraction. 3 rounds.
Second Week, 10 reps, 10 second Isometric contraction. 3 rounds.
Third Week, 30 reps, 30 second Isometric contraction. 2 rounds.

DAY ONE

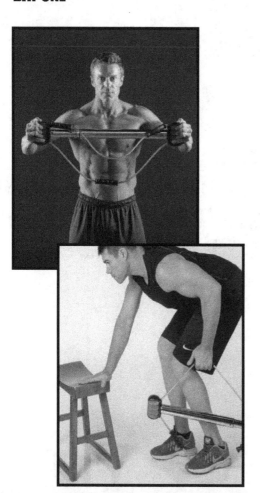

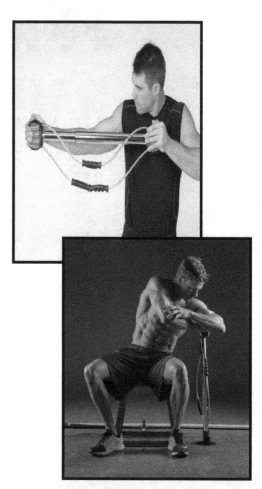

REP RANGE 20,10,30

08 REP RANGE PROGRAM

HOW TO PERFORM THIS ROUTINE:
First Week Perform 20 reps, 20 second Isometric contraction. 3 rounds.
Second Week, 10 reps, 10 second Isometric contraction. 3 rounds.
Third Week, 30 reps, 30 second Isometric contraction. 2 rounds.

DAY ONE continued.........

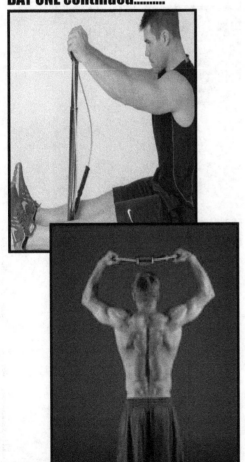

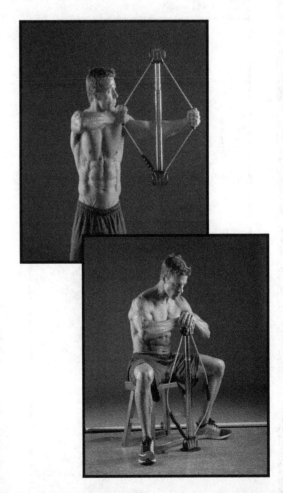

REP RANGE 20,10,30

08 REP RANGE PROGRAM

HOW TO PERFORM THIS ROUTINE:
First Week Perform 20 reps, 20 second Isometric contraction. 3 rounds.
Second Week, 10 reps, 10 second Isometric contraction. 3 rounds.
Third Week, 30 reps, 30 second Isometric contraction. 2 rounds.

DAY TWO

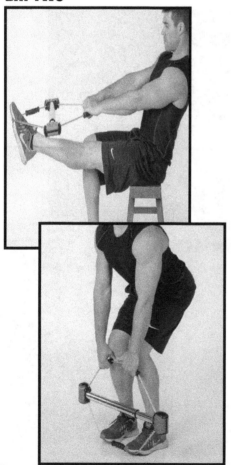

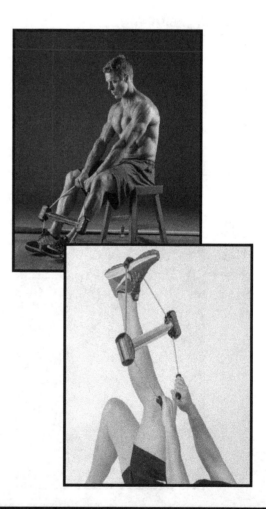

REP RANGE 20,10,30

08 REP RANGE PROGRAM

HOW TO PERFORM THIS ROUTINE:
First Week Perform 20 reps, 20 second Isometric contraction. 3 rounds.
Second Week, 10 reps, 10 second Isometric contraction. 3 rounds.
Third Week, 30 reps, 30 second Isometric contraction. 2 rounds.

DAY TWO continued............

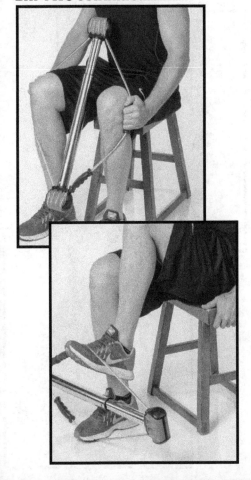

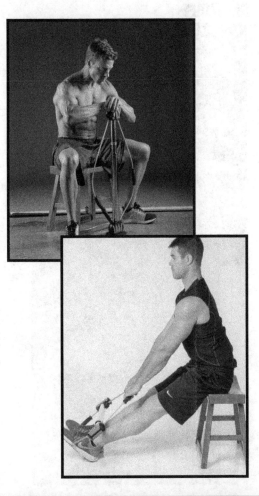

REP RANGE 20,10,30

08 REP RANGE PROGRAM

HOW TO PERFORM THIS ROUTINE:
First Week Perform 20 reps, 20 second Isometric contraction. 3 rounds.
Second Week, 10 reps, 10 second Isometric contraction. 3 rounds.
Third Week, 30 reps, 30 second Isometric contraction. 2 rounds.

DAY THREE

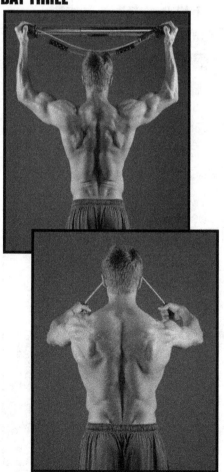

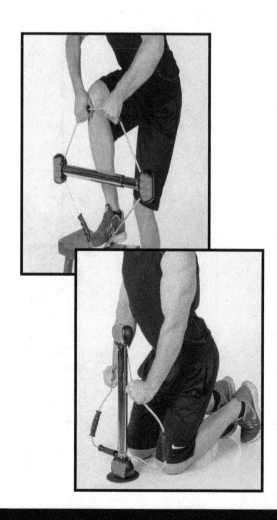

REP RANGE 20,10,30

08 REP RANGE PROGRAM

HOW TO PERFORM THIS ROUTINE:
First Week Perform 20 reps, 20 second Isometric contraction. 3 rounds.
Second Week, 10 reps, 10 second Isometric contraction. 3 rounds.
Third Week, 30 reps, 30 second Isometric contraction. 2 rounds.

DAY THREE continued.......

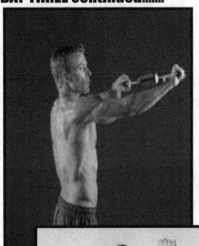
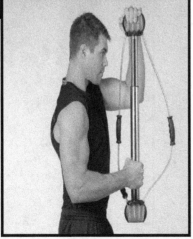
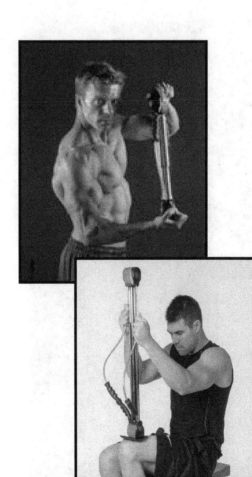

REP RANGE 20,10,30

08 REP RANGE PROGRAM

HOW TO PERFORM THIS ROUTINE:
First Week Perform 20 reps, 20 second Isometric contraction. 3 rounds.
Second Week, 10 reps, 10 second Isometric contraction. 3 rounds.
Third Week, 30 reps, 30 second Isometric contraction. 2 rounds.

DAY THREE continued.......

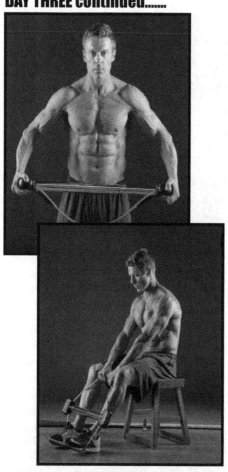
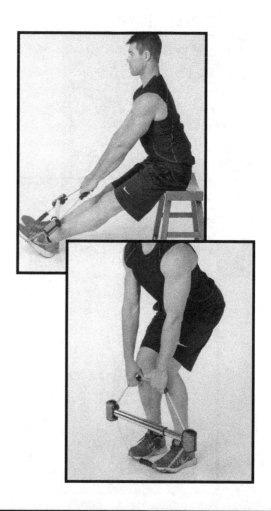

REP RANGE 20,10,30

08 REP RANGE PROGRAM

HOW TO PERFORM THIS ROUTINE:
First Week Perform 20 reps, 20 second Isometric contraction. 3 rounds.
Second Week, 10 reps, 10 second Isometric contraction. 3 rounds.
Third Week, 30 reps, 30 second Isometric contraction. 2 rounds.

DAY FOUR

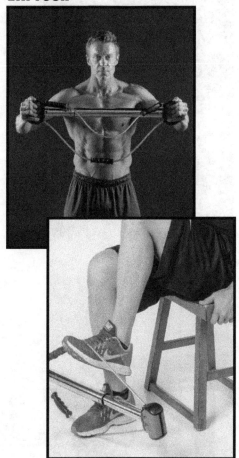

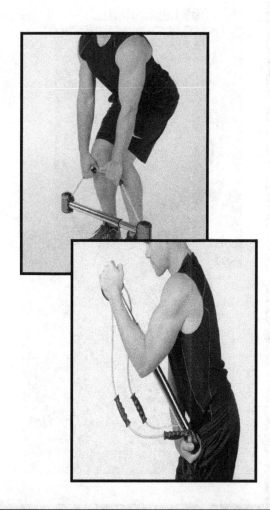

REP RANGE 20,10,30

08 REP RANGE PROGRAM

HOW TO PERFORM THIS ROUTINE:

First Week Perform 20 reps, 20 second Isometric contraction. 3 rounds.
Second Week, 10 reps, 10 second Isometric contraction. 3 rounds.
Third Week, 30 reps, 30 second Isometric contraction. 2 rounds.

DAY FOUR continued......

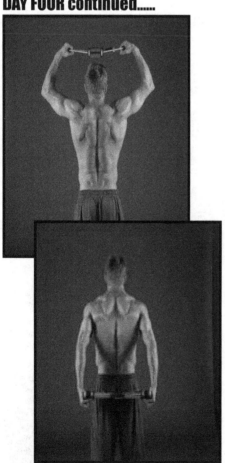

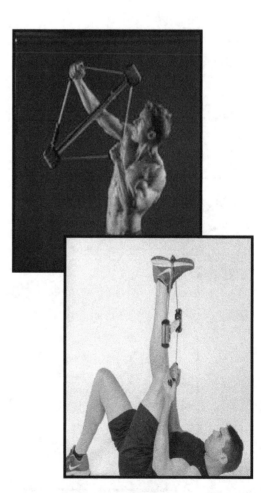

REP RANGE 20,10,30

08 REP RANGE PROGRAM

HOW TO PERFORM THIS ROUTINE:
First Week Perform 20 reps, 20 second Isometric contraction. 3 rounds.
Second Week, 10 reps, 10 second Isometric contraction. 3 rounds.
Third Week, 30 reps, 30 second Isometric contraction. 2 rounds.

DAY FIVE

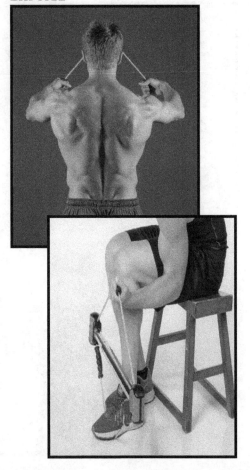

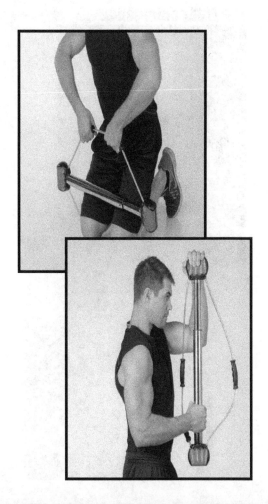

REP RANGE 20,10,30

08 REP RANGE PROGRAM

HOW TO PERFORM THIS ROUTINE:
First Week Perform 20 reps, 20 second Isometric contraction. 3 rounds.
Second Week, 10 reps, 10 second Isometric contraction. 3 rounds.
Third Week, 30 reps, 30 second Isometric contraction. 2 rounds.

DAY FIVE continued.....

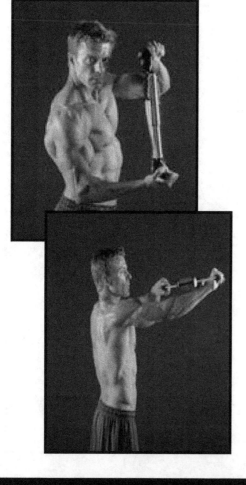

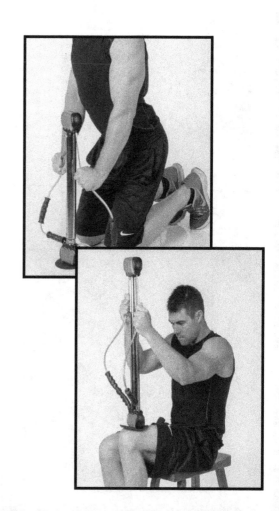

CHAPTER 9
REP RANGE
POWER 20 PROGRAM
PHASE 1
WEEK 1 OF 3
REP SPEED CONTRACT 1 SECOND, RELEASE 1 SECOND

REP RANGE POWER 20 PROGRAM

09 REP RANGE POWER 20 PROGRAM

REP RANGE POWER 20 PROGRAM " MUSCLE-BUILDING PHASE"

Phase 1: 25x20 Perform 25 reps followed by a 20 second isometric contraction. 2 sets per exercise

Phase 2: 15x20 Perform 15 reps followed by a 20 second isometric contraction. 2 sets per exercise.

Phase 3: 10x20 Perform 10 reps followed by a 20 second isometric contraction. 2 set per exercise

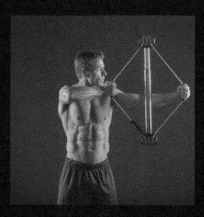

REP RANGE POWER 20 PROGRAM

09 REP RANGE POWER 20 PROGRAM

HOW TO PERFORM THIS ROUTINE:
PHASE ONE 25x20 PHASE
Perform 25 reps followed by a 20 second isometric contraction.
2 sets per exercise

DAY ONE

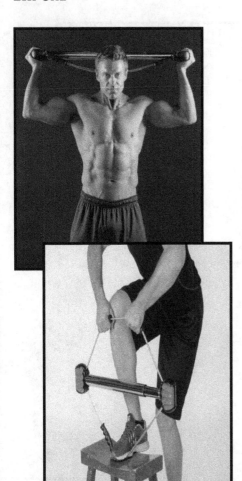
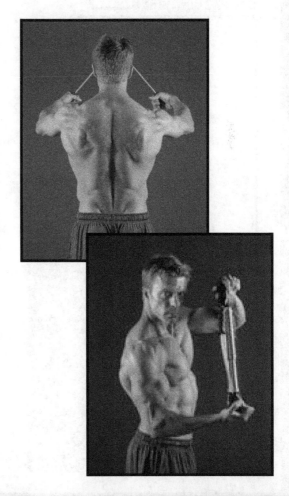

REP RANGE POWER 20 PROGRAM

09 REP RANGE POWER 20 PROGRAM

HOW TO PERFORM THIS ROUTINE:
PHASE ONE 25x20 PHASE

Perform 25 reps followed by a 20 second isometric contraction.
2 sets per exercise

DAY ONE continued...........

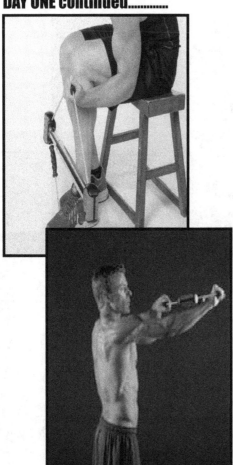

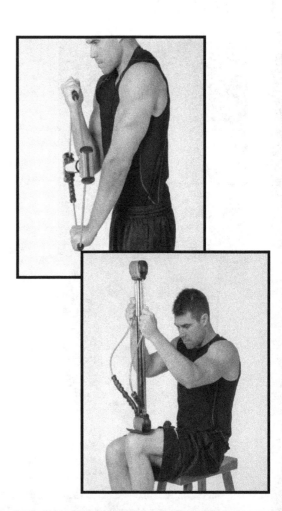

REP RANGE POWER 20 PROGRAM

09 REP RANGE POWER 20 PROGRAM

HOW TO PERFORM THIS ROUTINE:
PHASE ONE 25x20 PHASE
Perform 25 reps followed by a 20 second isometric contraction.
2 sets per exercise

DAY TWO

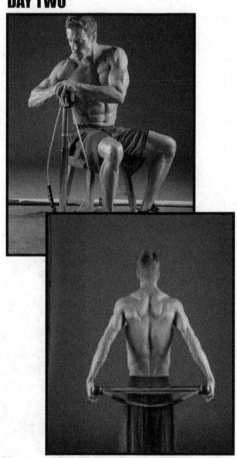

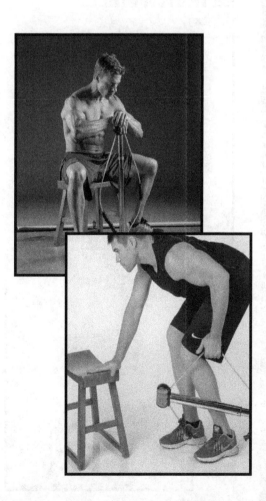

REP RANGE POWER 20 PROGRAM

09 REP RANGE POWER 20 PROGRAM

HOW TO PERFORM THIS ROUTINE:
PHASE ONE 25x20 PHASE

Perform 25 reps followed by a 20 second isometric contraction.
2 sets per exercise

DAY TWO continued.......

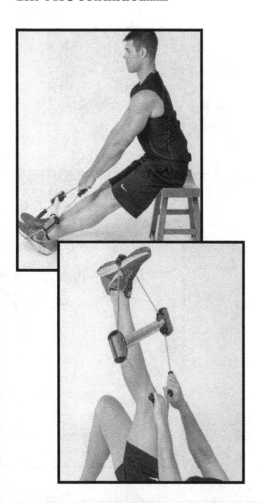

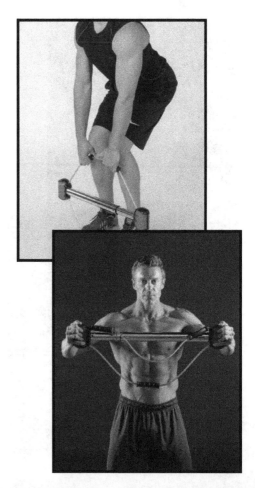

REP RANGE POWER 20 PROGRAM

09 REP RANGE POWER 20 PROGRAM

HOW TO PERFORM THIS ROUTINE:
PHASE ONE 25x20 PHASE

Perform 25 reps followed by a 20 second isometric contraction.
2 sets per exercise

DAY THREE

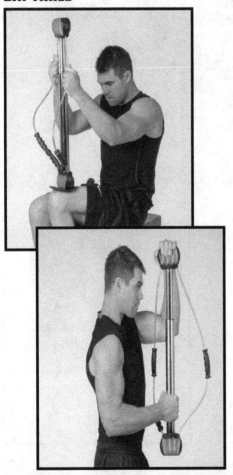

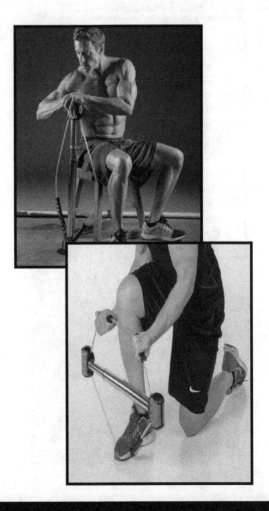

REP RANGE POWER 20 PROGRAM

09 REP RANGE POWER 20 PROGRAM

HOW TO PERFORM THIS ROUTINE:
PHASE ONE 25x20 PHASE

Perform 25 reps followed by a 20 second isometric contraction.
2 sets per exercise

DAY THREE continued..........

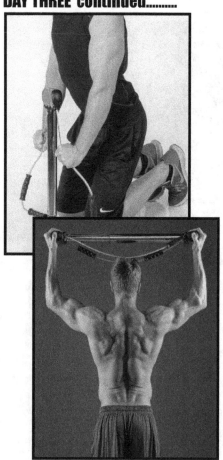

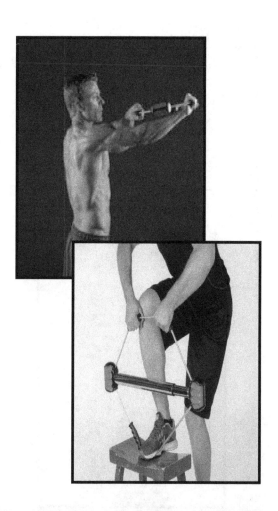

REP RANGE POWER 20 PROGRAM

09 REP RANGE POWER 20 PROGRAM

HOW TO PERFORM THIS ROUTINE:
PHASE ONE 25x20 PHASE

Perform 25 reps followed by a 20 second isometric contraction.
2 sets per exercise

DAY FOUR

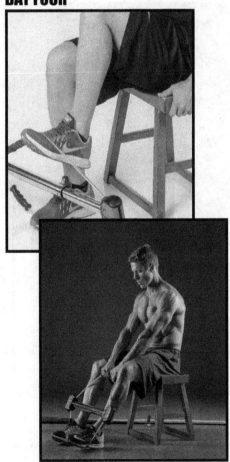

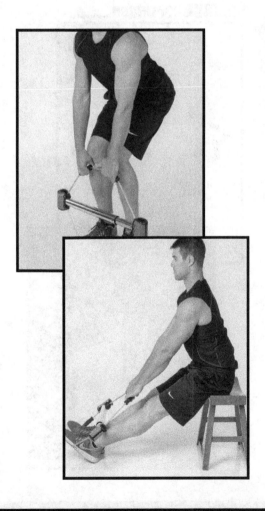

REP RANGE POWER 20 PROGRAM

09 REP RANGE POWER 20 PROGRAM

HOW TO PERFORM THIS ROUTINE:
PHASE ONE 25x20 PHASE

Perform 25 reps followed by a 20 second isometric contraction.
2 sets per exercise

DAY FOUR continued..........

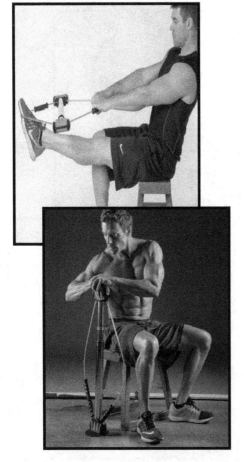

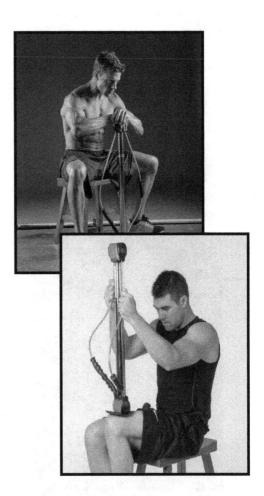

REP RANGE POWER 20 PROGRAM

09 REP RANGE POWER 20 PROGRAM

HOW TO PERFORM THIS ROUTINE:
PHASE ONE 25x20 PHASE
Perform 25 reps followed by a 20 second isometric contraction.
2 sets per exercise

DAY FIVE

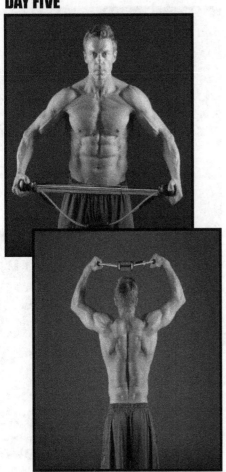

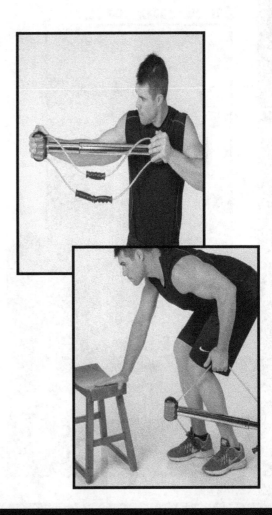

REP RANGE POWER 20 PROGRAM

09 REP RANGE POWER 20 PROGRAM

HOW TO PERFORM THIS ROUTINE:
PHASE ONE 25x20 PHASE

Perform 25 reps followed by a 20 second isometric contraction.
2 sets per exercise

DAY FIVE continued............

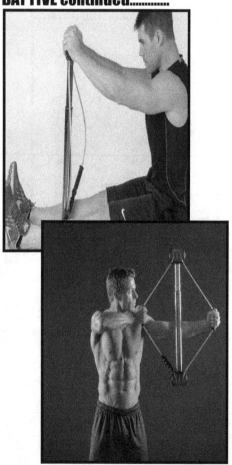

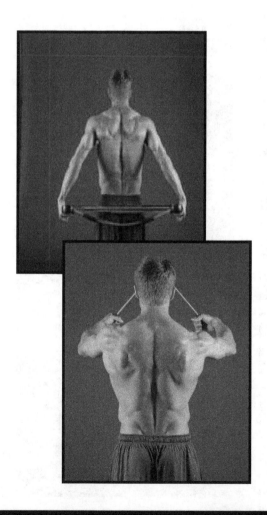

CHAPTER 9
REP RANGE
POWER 20 PROGRAM
PHASE 2
WEEK 2 OF 3
REP SPEED CONTRACT 1 SECOND, RELEASE 1 SECOND

REP RANGE POWER 20 PROGRAM

09 REP RANGE POWER 20 PROGRAM

HOW TO PERFORM THIS ROUTINE:
PHASE TWO 15x20 PHASE

Perform 15 reps followed by a 20 second isometric contraction.
2 sets per exercise

DAY ONE

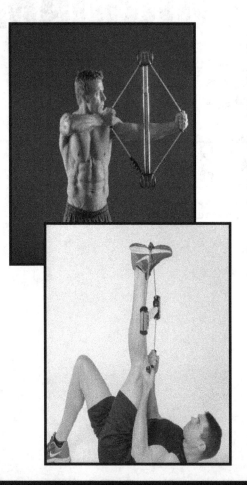
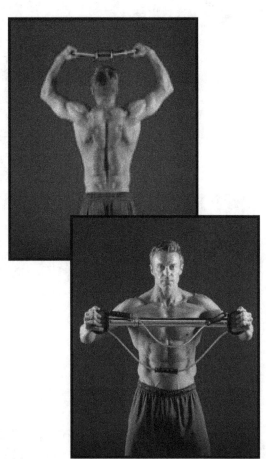

REP RANGE POWER 20 PROGRAM

09 REP RANGE POWER 20 PROGRAM

HOW TO PERFORM THIS ROUTINE:
PHASE TWO 15x20 PHASE

Perform 15 reps followed by a 20 second isometric contraction.
2 sets per exercise

DAY ONE continued..........

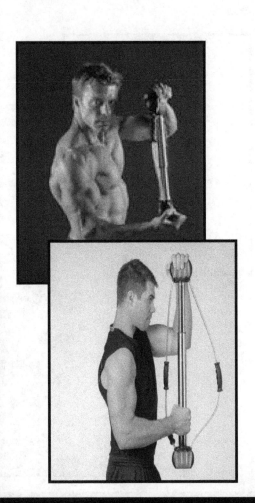

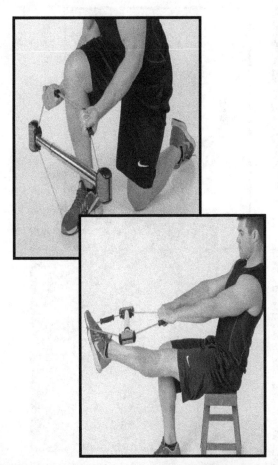

REP RANGE POWER 20 PROGRAM

09 REP RANGE POWER 20 PROGRAM

HOW TO PERFORM THIS ROUTINE:
PHASE TWO 15x20 PHASE

Perform 15 reps followed by a 20 second isometric contraction.
2 sets per exercise

DAY TWO

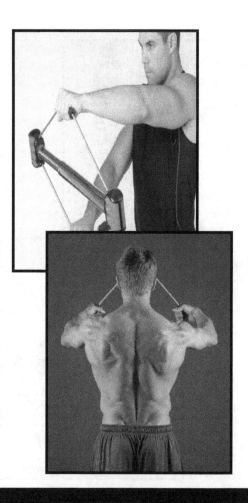
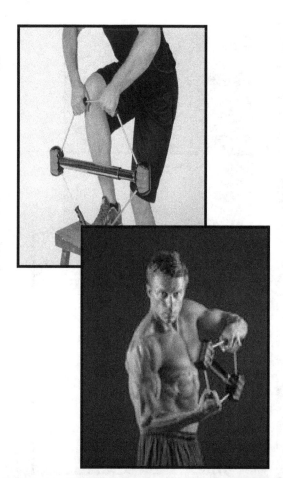

REP RANGE POWER 20 PROGRAM

09 REP RANGE POWER 20 PROGRAM

HOW TO PERFORM THIS ROUTINE:
PHASE TWO 15x20 PHASE

Perform 15 reps followed by a 20 second isometric contraction.
2 sets per exercise

DAY TWO continued.......

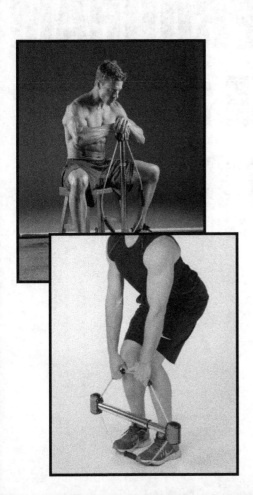

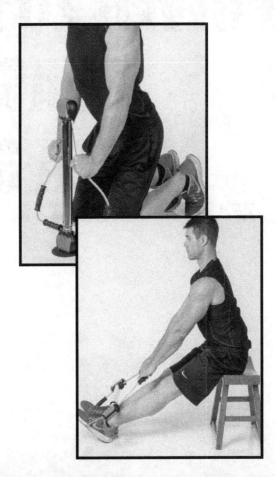

CHAPTER 9

REP RANGE

POWER 20 PROGRAM

PHASE 3

WEEK 3 OF 3

REP SPEED CONTRACT 1 SECOND, RELEASE 1 SECOND

REP RANGE POWER 20 PROGRAM

09 REP RANGE POWER 20 PROGRAM

HOW TO PERFORM THIS ROUTINE:
PHASE TWO 10x20 PHASE
Perform 10 reps followed by a 20 second isometric contraction.
2 sets per exercise

DAY ONE

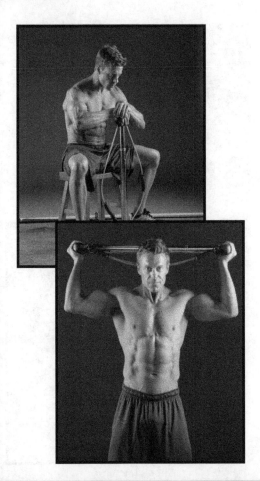

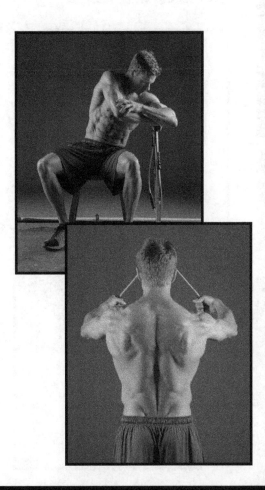

REP RANGE POWER 20 PROGRAM

09 REP RANGE POWER 20 PROGRAM

HOW TO PERFORM THIS ROUTINE:
PHASE THREE 10x20 PHASE
Perform 10 reps followed by a 20 second isometric contraction.
2 sets per exercise.

DAY ONE continued...........

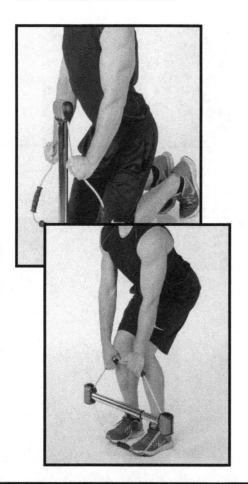

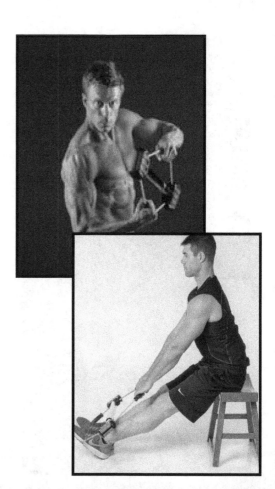

REP RANGE POWER 20 PROGRAM

09 REP RANGE POWER 20 PROGRAM

HOW TO PERFORM THIS ROUTINE:
PHASE THREE 10x20 PHASE

Perform 10 reps followed by a 20 second isometric contraction.
2 sets per exercise.

DAY TWO

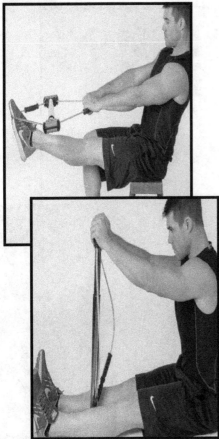

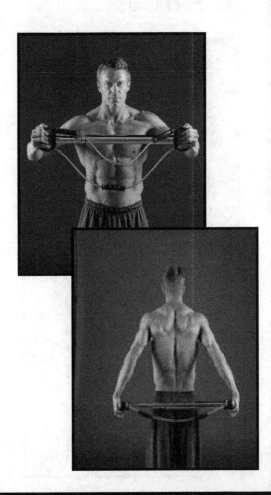

REP RANGE POWER 20 PROGRAM

09 REP RANGE POWER 20 PROGRAM

HOW TO PERFORM THIS ROUTINE:
PHASE THREE 10x20 PHASE
Perform 10 reps followed by a 20 second isometric contraction.
2 sets per exercise.

DAY TWO continued..........

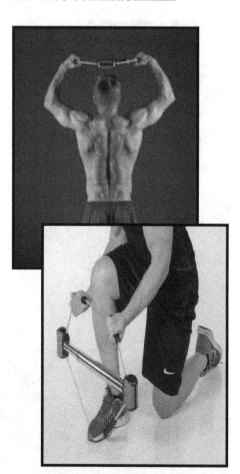

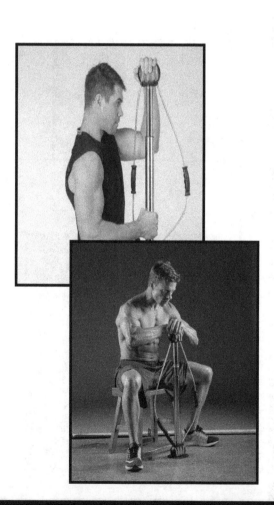

CHAPTER 10

REP RANGE

ISO-POWER 10

PHASE 13

PERFORM 10 REPS, EACH REP IS HELD FOR 10 SECONDS

THE ISO-POWER 10 PROGRAM

10 THE ISO-POWER 10 PROGRAM

HOW TO PERFORM THIS ROUTINE:
THE ISO-POWER 10 PROGRAM

Perform the **POWER 10 WORKOUT**—by performing 10 reps. Each rep is held for 10 seconds. Perform all exercises one after the other until all exercises are completed without rest. Perform 3 rounds of these between each round rest for 5 seconds before starting the round again.
Alternate day one and day two for 6 days per week.
DAY ONE

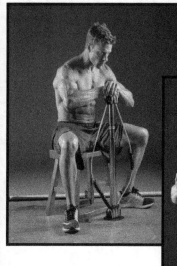
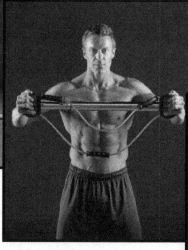
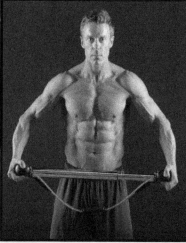

THE ISO-POWER 10 PROGRAM

10 THE ISO-POWER 10 PROGRAM

HOW TO PERFORM THIS ROUTINE:
THE ISO-POWER 10 PROGRAM

Perform the **POWER 10 WORKOUT**—by performing 10 reps. Each rep is held for 10 seconds. Perform all exercises one after the other until all exercises are completed without rest. Perform 3 rounds of these between each round rest for 5 seconds before starting the round again.
Alternate day one and day two for 6 days per week.
DAY ONE continued..........

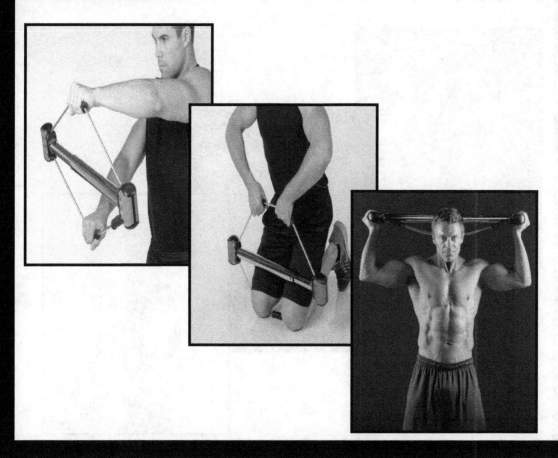

THE ISO-POWER 10 PROGRAM

10 THE ISO-POWER 10 PROGRAM

HOW TO PERFORM THIS ROUTINE:
THE ISO-POWER 10 PROGRAM

Perform the **POWER 10 WORKOUT**—by performing 10 reps. Each rep is held for 10 seconds. Perform all exercises one after the other until all exercises are completed without rest. Perform 3 rounds of these between each round rest for 5 seconds before starting the round again.
Alternate day one and day two for 6 days per week.
DAY ONE continued......

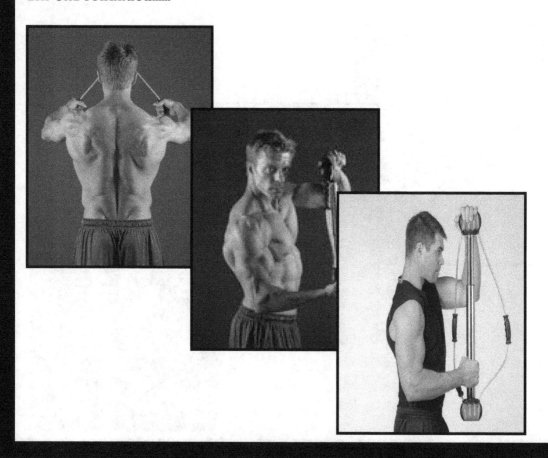

THE ISO-POWER 10 PROGRAM

10 THE ISO-POWER 10 PROGRAM

HOW TO PERFORM THIS ROUTINE:
THE ISO-POWER 10 PROGRAM

Perform the **POWER 10 WORKOUT**—by performing 10 reps. Each rep is held for 10 seconds. Perform all exercises one after the other until all exercises are completed without rest. Perform 3 rounds of these between each round rest for 5 seconds before starting the round again.
Alternate day one and day two for 6 days per week.
DAY TWO

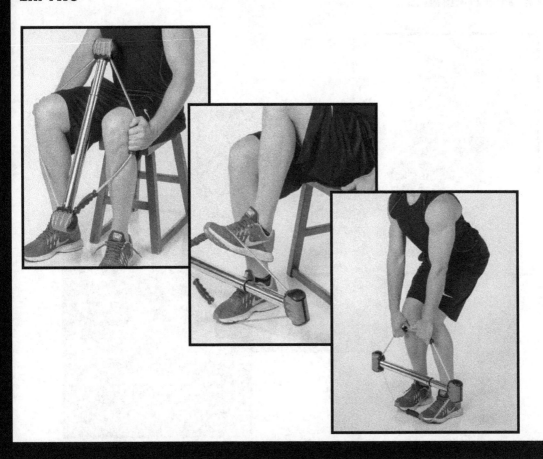

THE ISO-POWER 10 PROGRAM

10 THE ISO-POWER 10 PROGRAM

HOW TO PERFORM THIS ROUTINE:
THE ISO-POWER 10 PROGRAM

Perform the **POWER 10 WORKOUT**—by performing 10 reps. Each rep is held for 10 seconds. Perform all exercises one after the other until all exercises are completed without rest. Perform 3 rounds of these between each round rest for 5 seconds before starting the round again.
Alternate day one and day two for 6 days per week.
DAY TWO continue........

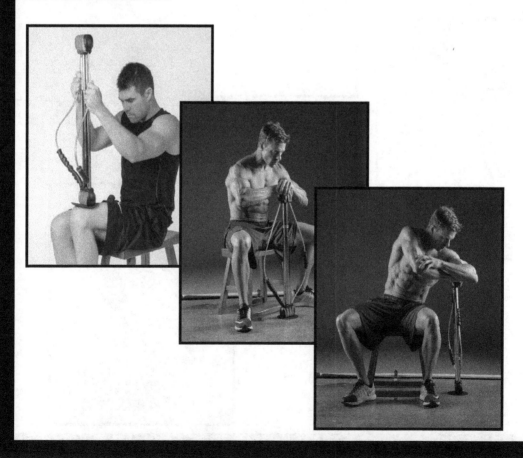

THE ISO-POWER 10 PROGRAM

10 THE ISO-POWER 10 PROGRAM

HOW TO PERFORM THIS ROUTINE:
THE ISO-POWER 10 PROGRAM

Perform the **POWER 10 WORKOUT**—by performing 10 reps. Each rep is held for 10 seconds. Perform all exercises one after the other until all exercises are completed without rest. Perform 3 rounds of these between each round rest for 5 seconds before starting the round again.
Alternate day one and day two for 6 days per week.
DAY TWO continued...........

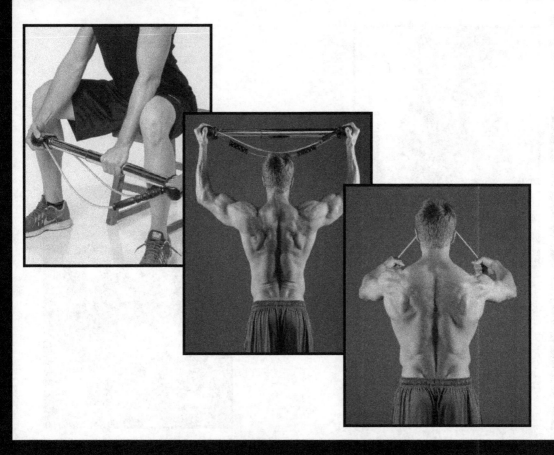

THE ISO-POWER 10 PROGRAM

10 THE ISO-POWER 10 PROGRAM

HOW TO PERFORM THIS ROUTINE:
THE ISO-POWER 10 PROGRAM

Perform the **POWER 10 WORKOUT**—by performing 10 reps. Each rep is held for 10 seconds. Perform all exercises one after the other until all exercises are completed without rest. Perform 3 rounds of these between each round rest for 5 seconds before starting the round again.
Alternate day one and day two for 6 days per week.
DAY TWO continued...........

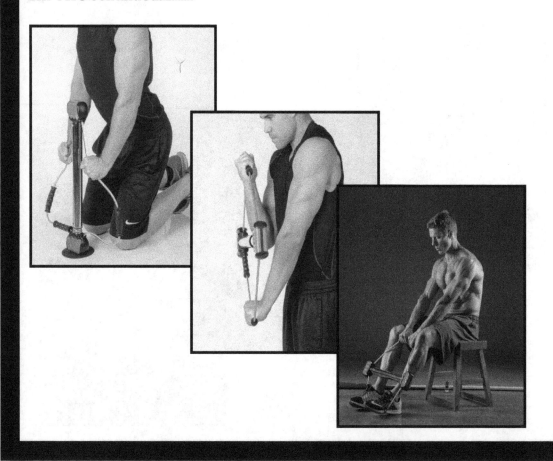

CHAPTER 11
POWER REP WEEK
ISO-POWER FREESTYLE
PHASE ONE

REP RANGES CHANGE THROUGHOUT THE WEEK

ISO-POWER FREESTYLE PROGRAM

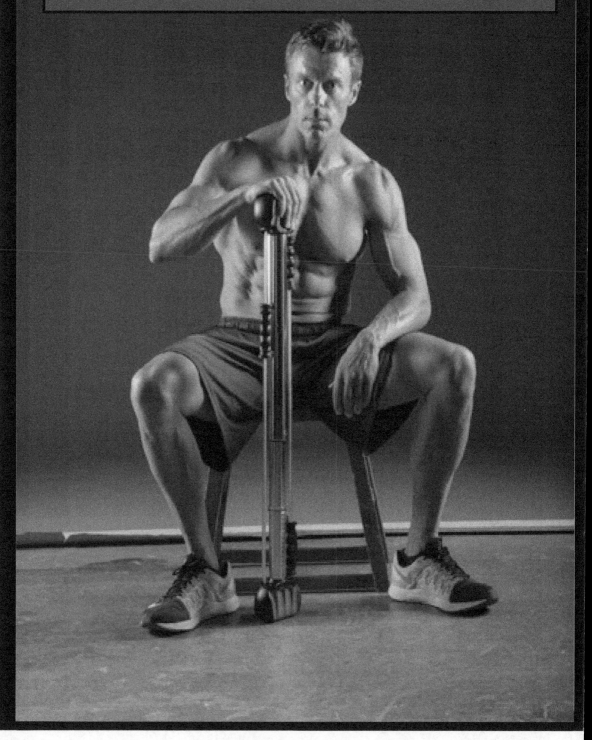

ISO-POWER FREESTYLE PROGRAM

11 ISO-POWER FREESTYLE PROGRAM PHASE ONE

HOW TO PERFORM THIS ROUTINE:
ISO-POWER FREESTYLE PROGRAM

Day 1=20 reps, Day 2=15 reps, Day 3=10 reps, Day 4=25 reps, Day 5=15 reps
Day 6=30 reps, Day 7=10 reps. On the last rep perform a 20 second
Isometric contraction. Perform all exercises without rest for 2 rounds.
Perform this routine every day 7 days per week for 3 weeks

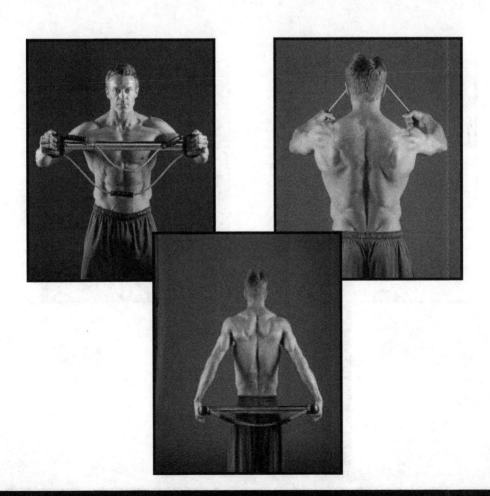

ISO-POWER FREESTYLE PROGRAM

11 ISO-POWER FREESTYLE PROGRAM PHASE ONE

HOW TO PERFORM THIS ROUTINE:
ISO-POWER FREESTYLE PROGRAM

Day 1=20 reps, Day 2=15 reps, Day 3=10 reps, Day 4=25 reps, Day 5=15 reps
Day 6=30 reps, Day 7=10 reps. On the last rep perform a 20 second
Isometric contraction. Perform all exercises without rest for 2 rounds.
Perform this routine every day 7 days per week for 3 weeks

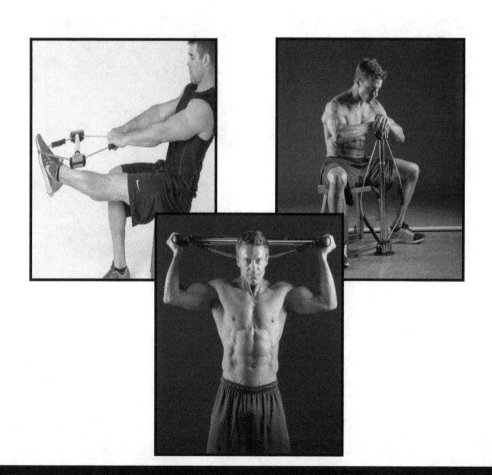

ISO-POWER FREESTYLE PROGRAM

11 ISO-POWER FREESTYLE PROGRAM PHASE ONE

HOW TO PERFORM THIS ROUTINE:
ISO-POWER FREESTYLE PROGRAM

Day 1=20 reps, Day 2=15 reps, Day 3=10 reps, Day 4=25 reps, Day 5=15 reps
Day 6=30 reps, Day 7=10 reps. On the last rep perform a 20 second
Isometric contraction. Perform all exercises without rest for 2 rounds.
Perform this routine every day 7 days per week for 3 weeks

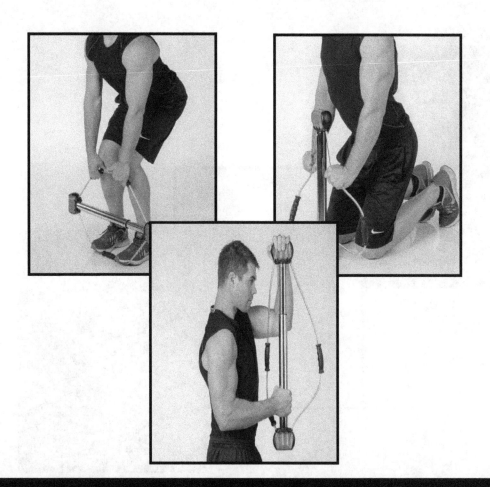

PHASE TWO

11 ISO-POWER FREESTYLE PROGRAM PHASE TWO

HOW TO PERFORM THIS ROUTINE:
THE ISO-POWER FREESTYLE PROGRAM

Day 1=10 reps, Day 2=10 reps, Day 3=7 reps, Day 4=15 reps, Day 5=10 reps
Day 6=20 reps, Day 7=5 reps. On the last rep perform a 30 second
Isometric contraction. Perform all exercises without rest for 2 rounds.
Perform this routine every day 7 days per week for 3 weeks

DAY ONE

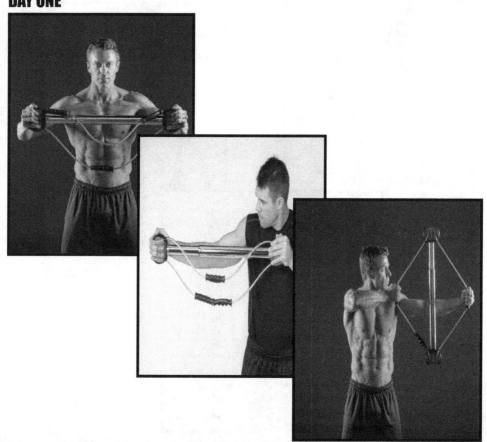

PHASE TWO

11 ISO-POWER FREESTYLE PROGRAM PHASE TWO

HOW TO PERFORM THIS ROUTINE:
THE ISO-POWER FREESTYLE PROGRAM

Day 1=10 reps, Day 2=10 reps, Day 3=7 reps, Day 4=15 reps, Day 5=10 reps
Day 6=20 reps, Day 7=5 reps. On the last rep perform a 30 second
Isometric contraction. Perform all exercises without rest for 2 rounds.
Perform this routine every day 7 days per week for 3 weeks

DAY ONE continued..........

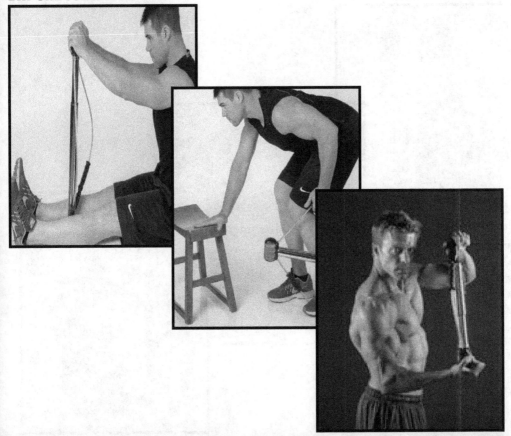

PHASE TWO

11 ISO-POWER FREESTYLE PROGRAM PHASE TWO

HOW TO PERFORM THIS ROUTINE:
THE ISO-POWER FREESTYLE PROGRAM

Day 1=10 reps, Day 2=10 reps, Day 3=7 reps, Day 4=15 reps, Day 5=10 reps
Day 6=20 reps, Day 7=5 reps. On the last rep perform a 30 second
Isometric contraction. Perform all exercises without rest for 2 rounds.
Perform this routine every day 7 days per week for 3 weeks

DAY ONE contin........

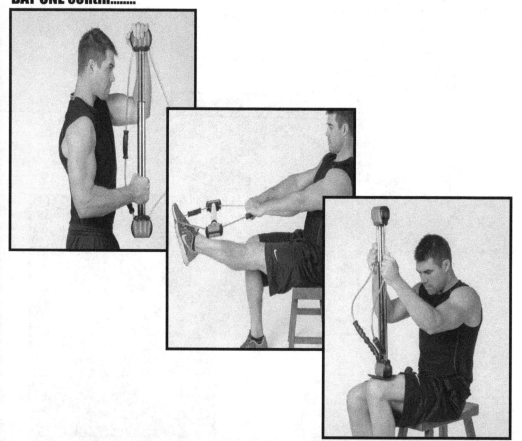

PHASE TWO

11 ISO-POWER FREESTYLE PROGRAM PHASE TWO

HOW TO PERFORM THIS ROUTINE:
THE ISO-POWER FREESTYLE PROGRAM

Day 1=10 reps, Day 2=10 reps, Day 3=7 reps, Day 4=15 reps, Day 5=10 reps
Day 6=20 reps, Day 7=5 reps. On the last rep perform a 30 second
Isometric contraction. Perform all exercises without rest for 2 rounds.
Perform this routine every day 7 days per week for 3 weeks

DAY TWO

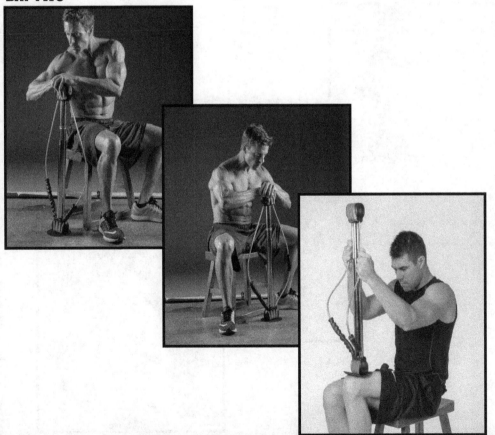

PHASE TWO

11 ISO-POWER FREESTYLE PROGRAM PHASE TWO

HOW TO PERFORM THIS ROUTINE:
THE ISO-POWER FREESTYLE PROGRAM

Day 1=10 reps, Day 2=10 reps, Day 3=7 reps, Day 4=15 reps, Day 5=10 reps
Day 6=20 reps, Day 7=5 reps. On the last rep perform a 30 second
Isometric contraction. Perform all exercises without rest for 2 rounds.
Perform this routine every day 7 days per week for 3 weeks

DAY TWO continued...........

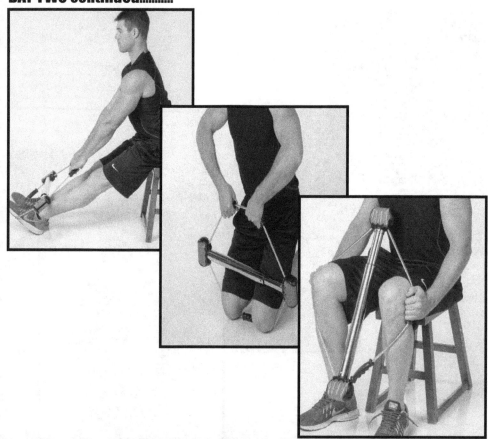

PHASE TWO

11 ISO-POWER FREESTYLE PROGRAM PHASE TWO

HOW TO PERFORM THIS ROUTINE:
THE ISO-POWER FREESTYLE PROGRAM

Day 1=10 reps, Day 2=10 reps, Day 3=7 reps, Day 4=15 reps, Day 5=10 reps
Day 6=20 reps, Day 7=5 reps. On the last rep perform a 30 second
Isometric contraction. Perform all exercises without rest for 2 rounds.
Perform this routine every day 7 days per week for 3 weeks

DAY TWO continued...........

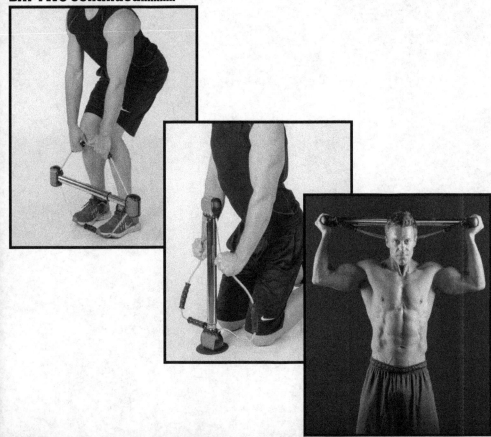

Looking forward to hearing from you on your progress. Please drop me an email skippymarl@icloud.com

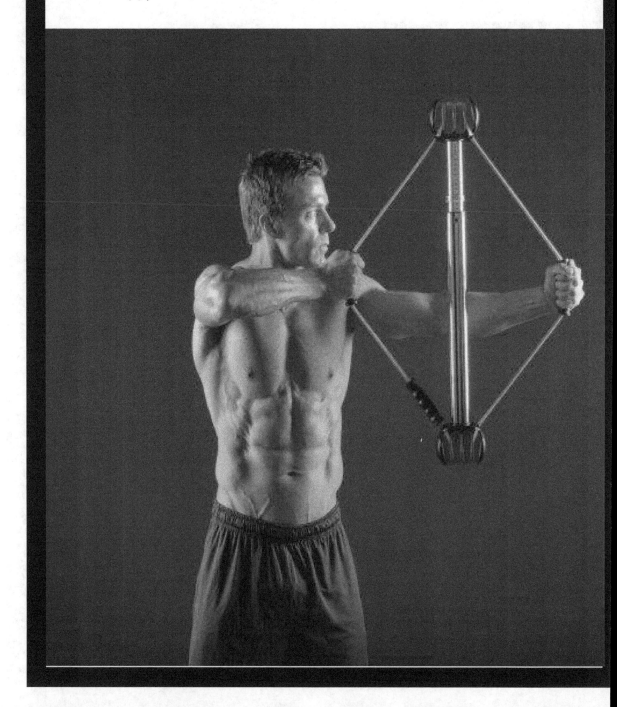

MOST IMPROVED STUDENT AWARD
COMING SOON
SEPTEMBER 15th 2019

CPSIA information can be obtained
at www.ICGtesting.com
Printed in the USA
BVHW061829090919
557952BV00011B/1177/P

9 781927 558867